The Transgender Self-Care Journal

The TRANSGENDER SELF-CARE JOURNAL

Prompts and Practices to Care for Your **BEAUTIFUL SELF**

Andrew Maxwell Triska, LCSW

ROCKRIDGE
PRESS

Interior and Cover Designer: Jane Archer
Art Producer: Sara Feinstein
Editor: Adrian Potts
Production Editor: Ruth Sakata Corley
Production Manager: Jose Olivera
Author photo courtesy of Peter O'Loghlen

ISBN: Print 978-1-64876-318-2
R0

CONTENTS

"A friend taught me:
your life's work begins
where your great joy meets
the world's great hunger."

—*Kate Bornstein*

INTRODUCTION

Thanks for picking up *The Transgender Self-Care Journal.* This journal is a space for you to develop your self-care skills and improve your ability to prioritize your own needs. Journals can be helpful to record thoughts that you might otherwise forget, to explore feelings you haven't delved into very deeply, or to go back and re-examine the way your feelings have changed about something.

You might have negative associations with the term "self-care." Maybe it's linked in your mind with overpriced bath bombs and way-too-cheerful self-help gurus. And it's true that the concept of self-care can be toxic when it's misused to blame people for their own mental health struggles, replace professional treatment, or sell consumer goods. It's also true that self-care is sometimes promoted as a way to increase your productivity, as though caring for yourself is only important if it helps you perform better at your job or advance your career. However, true self-care—at its core—is about recognizing and attending to your own needs.

It's easy to mistake self-care for a set of things you *do*, like going to the gym or taking a spa day. But more than anything, self-care is about the *beliefs* you have about the value of your wants, needs, and feelings. Sometimes, without even thinking about it, you might find yourself taking other people's problems more seriously than your own. Have you ever picked up an extra shift at work because you were afraid your coworker would be upset if you didn't? Have you ever found yourself doing all the housework when your partner didn't feel like it? Do you ever think, "I need support, but I shouldn't bother my friends"? Self-care means responding to situations like these in a way that treats your needs as important.

Why is self-care so important if you're trans? As a trans-identified psychotherapist whose practice focuses on queer and trans mental health, I've seen more clients than I can count who consistently put their needs last. Maybe you feel like your identity makes you less deserving of help. Maybe you think you have to be twice as good as other people to get recognized. Or maybe the stress of being a gender minority layered on top of other life stressors has become too much to handle.

This journal contains prompts, exercises, affirmations, and quotes to help you get to a better place with true self-care—recognizing your needs and attending to them. In this journal, you'll be asked to delve deeper into what you're feeling, how you relate to your emotions, and what your habits around your needs look like. If you're feeling tired or stressed on a particular day, you'll be asked to take a look at why those feelings exist and what factors you can control. Conversely, if you're feeling great one day, you can reflect on why that day is different from other days.

While this journal is a great way to gain insight into feelings like sadness, anxiety, and guilt, it's not a substitute for a therapist. The resources section has info about how to find trans-competent therapy. You might find that after getting your thoughts down on paper, you've gained more clarity about your needs and are ready to seek therapy. This journal can also be helpful if you already see a therapist and would like to record your thoughts between sessions.

With that in mind, let's jump into the first part of this book, where you'll take a closer look at your thoughts and emotions.

Nurture Your Mind

It's tough to care for yourself when you're not even sure how you're feeling or what you need. Some people find it difficult to recognize or name their emotions, even to themselves. Or you may be able to describe emotions like sadness, or physical sensations like fatigue, without being able to connect them to anything that's going on in your life. Many trans people experience so much invalidation that it can be hard for them to trust themselves.

This section is all about self-reflection: getting in touch with your feelings, however clichéd that sounds. Here, you'll turn vague memories and indistinct body sensations into more concrete descriptions of how you're feeling and what's causing it. Prompts, exercises, affirmations, and quotes in this section will focus on creating a base of self-awareness on which you can build self-care.

"In running from anxiety you lose your most precious opportunities for the emergence of yourself, and for your education as a human being."

—*Rollo May*

Sometimes, emotions can cause physical sensations in your body. Anxiety might make your stomach hurt or give you a headache. Joy can make you feel lighter. Write about some physical sensations of emotion that you've experienced in the past week.

Taking a Pause

Close your eyes, lie down on a comfortable surface, and spend five minutes doing a full-body scan from the top of your head to your feet. Try to notice things like muscle tension, chest tightness, or any other discomfort. Don't try to relax or control these sensations—just observe them. When you're finished, reflect on what you noticed. Pain, hunger, tension? Signs you might need to rest, eat something, or take a walk? This week, try to get into the habit of stopping for a moment, paying attention, and responding to your body's signals.

When asked to describe their emotions, some people relay thoughts or events instead. Their answer to "How are you feeling?" might be "Someone misgendered me at work today" or "I'm feeling like I need a vacation" (thoughts) instead of "I'm feeling angry" or "I'm sad" (emotions). If you can't recognize or name your emotions, you might make decisions without fully understanding why you're making them. Write about a time you experienced intense emotion this week—without describing what happened or your opinion. Instead, write about the emotions you felt during the event.

Self-advocacy comes from self-awareness. If you build your self-awareness, you can learn to recognize your needs and ask for the things you want. Write about a time when you were scared to ask for something but were glad you did it anyway.

_____

_____

_____

_____

_____

_____

_____

_____

_____

_____

_____

_____

_____

_____

_____

The phrase "locus of control" refers to the sense of control you feel over your life. People with a more *external* locus tend to feel like their lives are dictated by other people, circumstances, or random chance. People with a more *internal* locus feel like they're the ones in control—but this can cause anxiety, as they may feel responsible for things outside their control, like other people's behavior. Write about your locus of control and how it's affected you.

If you've been invalidated in the past, it can be hard to see your feelings as real or trustworthy. Write about a time you convinced yourself to ignore your feelings and what the consequences were. Add a sentence or two about what could have happened if you had trusted and listened to yourself.

_____

_____

_____

_____

_____

_____

_____

_____

_____

_____

_____

_____

_____

I don't always have to know exactly what I'm thinking and feeling. It's okay if my thoughts are confused or vague. I can take my time learning how to identify and communicate my feelings to others.

What beliefs do you have about emotion? Some people feel bad about having or talking about negative emotions. You might feel that you're bringing more negativity into the world, or that acknowledging an emotion will make it worse. However, ignoring negative emotions doesn't make them go away, and adding a layer of shame and guilt won't make you feel any better. Identifying your emotions is the first step to understanding the beliefs, behaviors, and situations that cause them. Write about a negative emotion you've experienced—without judging or trying to dispel that emotion.

Sometimes, the way we identify or experience our emotions is interpreted based on gender stereotypes. You might be called feminine if you're sad or cry easily, or masculine if you get angry or raise your voice. This may make you uncomfortable expressing the "wrong" emotions for your identified or expressed gender. Write about a stereotype that has affected the way you express emotion.

Have you felt anxious and on edge lately? Anxiety has been described as a combination of hope and fear: a sense that things might get better combined with the fear that you won't be able to make that happen. If you didn't have anything to look forward to, you wouldn't be anxious. What hopes does your anxiety reflect?

_____

_____

_____

_____

_____

_____

_____

_____

_____

_____

_____

_____

_____

How do you usually describe the things that happen to you? Some people focus more on concrete details than on their inner experiences when reflecting on an event. This can make it difficult to think or talk about the meaning of events in your life. Write about a significant event in your life, but focus on the emotions you felt during the event rather than the physical details.

Knowing Your Values

Feelings of discomfort or unhappiness often have to do with our core values. When you're going against one of your values—for example, if you value honesty and openness, but you're doing something you see as inauthentic—you might feel a sense of unease. If you're not in touch with your values, you might not know where that feeling is coming from.

Circle any word that represents one of your values. Feel free to add some of your own.

family

compassion

friendship

faith

learning

responsibility

pleasure

art

beauty

generosity

self-reliance

justice

freedom

challenge

truth

ethics

self-improvement

happiness

service

stability

productivity

knowledge

health

order

adventure

_____

_____

_____

_____

_____

_____

_____

At some point in your life, you may have said something like "I always screw things up" or "I never get a break." This is called "overgeneralization": interpreting unrelated events as a universal rule.

In the following spaces, turn overgeneralizations into more realistic interpretations.

Example:

People always let me down → *I've had bad experiences, but I've always had one or two friends I could trust.*

_____ → _____

_____ → _____

_____ → _____

_____ → _____

_____ → _____

_____ → _____

Have you ever jumped to conclusions about what other people were thinking? Maybe you've thought something like "That woman stared at me, so she must think I'm ugly and weird" or "I'm sure people are just being nice to me when they say they see me as a man." This is called "mind reading": being certain about what other people feel or think without any evidence. Write about a time you mind read in the last few months and how it made you feel.

_____

_____

_____

_____

_____

_____

_____

_____

_____

_____

_____

_____

Sometimes, you might catch yourself thinking with your feelings. For example, you might think to yourself, "I feel bad, therefore I must have done something bad." Or, "I'm anxious, which means bad things will happen." Write about any strong feelings you've had lately. What thoughts have they prompted?

Some people feel like they can't move forward unless they feel 100 percent certain about what they're about to do, even if it's a small decision. With big decisions—like moving cities, or having gender-affirming medical treatment—fear of uncertainty can be paralyzing. However, learning to tolerate the emotions that come with uncertainty can help you keep going when you feel stuck. In the following space, write about your relationship with uncertainty and how it's affected your life. Observe any feelings that arise, and allow them to come and go without judgment.

Decatastrophizing

Do you catastrophize? Catastrophizing means assuming that the worst will happen—for example, that coming out as trans at work means you'll be fired. If any of these are true about you, you might be prone to catastrophizing:

○ I spend days immobilized by indecision.

○ Friends say I assume the worst about people.

○ It's sometimes hard to define exactly what I'm worried about.

○ I catch myself thinking of unlikely scenarios, like friends suddenly turning on me.

○ When I think carefully, I realize there's no evidence for the awful scenarios I worry about.

○ Often, the worst-case scenarios I worry about aren't so bad when they actually happen.

You can often ease your anxiety by doing something called "decatastrophizing." First, think about the absolute worst-case scenario that could come from a given decision (e.g., "If I choose the wrong job, my life will be horrible."). Second, assess how likely this scenario is to occur (e.g., "Even if this job isn't everything I want, I'm 95 percent sure it won't be bad enough to make my *entire life* horrible."). Third, think about how you'd handle it if it *did* happen (e.g., "If it turned out to be the wrong job for me, I'd start applying for other jobs or see if I could go back to my old job.").

Have you ever felt like you complained too much about your life or the people around you? Complaints often reflect unmet needs that are larger than a single annoyance. Uncovering the larger needs behind small complaints can make it easier to have bigger, more comprehensive conversations about your needs or to make changes that don't just put a Band-Aid on your problems. In the following space, turn your complaints into needs.

Examples:

My partner spent too much money this weekend. → *I need consistency and stability.*

My boss didn't acknowledge my successful project. → *I need appreciation for my work.*

_____ → _____

_____ → _____

_____ → _____

_____ → _____

_____ → _____

_____ → _____

Write about a time you felt seen. It could be by someone in your life, a passage from a book, or even a cartoon.

_____

_____

_____

_____

_____

_____

_____

_____

_____

_____

_____

_____

_____

_____

_____

_____

Write about a moment of clarity you've had about your identity or values in life. What made that moment so meaningful?

_____

_____

_____

_____

_____

_____

_____

_____

_____

_____

_____

_____

_____

_____

Sitting with Your Feelings

Some people hesitate to identify their emotions because they believe they need to *do* something about every emotion they feel. You might feel, for example, like being angry at someone means you automatically have to confront them. Think of an emotion that you don't particularly want to act on. Sit and think about that emotion for the next two minutes, but without trying to think up a solution to it. Rate the strength of the emotion at the beginning and end of the exercise on a scale of 1 to 10. Learning to feel strong emotions without acting on them can be good practice if:

- You act on impulse in response to strong feelings.

- You deal with hurt or rejection by lashing out.

- You tell yourself you "shouldn't" have an emotion if there's no concrete way you can or should act on it.

- You feel ashamed because you equate feeling strong emotions with "losing control."

- Your negative emotions sometimes feel so strong that you fear you'll never feel better.

Sometimes, major life changes—like graduating from college or retiring—can cause you to rethink the purpose of your life. Questions like "What do I want?" and "What is life for?" might start to surface. While these thoughts might be overwhelming, they can also provide the impetus to make meaningful changes. After all, it's better to realize that you need to change course now than to stay on a path that isn't making you happy. Write about a major life transition you've experienced and what questions it brought up for you.

Build Your Inner Strength

Just by being a person with a trans identity—whether you're open about it or not—you've committed to being bold and adventurous in many large and small ways. You may not feel ready for acts of bravery just yet—in fact, you may feel annoyed that you even *have* to be brave. Like it or not, bravery comes with the territory. Existing as a trans person in the world means questioning norms, challenging stereotypes, and being a relentless self-advocate.

This section is all about facing down anxiety, coping with difficult emotions, and building your capacity to withstand adversity. Prompts, exercises, affirmations, and quotes in this section will center on understanding your own capacities and assembling an arsenal of emotional tools that will allow you to survive the challenges of your future.

"We feel like we know trans people if we just follow them on Instagram . . . What I'm always trying to do with my art is not just sort of say, 'Trans people deserve rights,' but rather, 'Trans people are emotionally complex, confused, loving, hating, depressed, wonderful, exquisite, boring.'"

—Alok Vaid-Menon

Good Vibes Only?

Have you ever been told to "think positive" when you were feeling crappy? Or that you need to "be grateful" or "change your perspective" about serious problems? These are examples of what's called "toxic positivity": the idea that feeling sad or anxious is unacceptable, or that you can change these emotions by sheer force of will. There's nothing wrong with being an optimist, even in the face of daunting challenges. However, toxic positivity can make you feel ashamed or inadequate about the normal ups and downs of life.

If you check more than one of these items, you might be suffering from toxic positivity:

○ I'm worried that if I talk about my problems, people will think I'm a downer.

○ I shouldn't be unhappy because other people have it worse.

○ I look much happier on social media than I am in real life.

○ I avoid thinking about negative emotions at all costs.

○ People in my life invalidate my feelings when they're not positive.

○ I've been told that happiness is just a matter of perspective.

Many people with gender identities that differ from the norm feel like they're somehow burdening others. Maybe you've been told that your transition is difficult for your family, or that making people use they/them pronouns at work is unreasonable. This might make you feel less likely to make yourself heard in other situations. Write about a time when you felt that you couldn't voice your needs to others.

I have the right to feel angry sometimes. No one can tell me that my anger or frustration is not valid. I have choices in how to express my anger, but I will not tell myself not to experience anger at all.

Write about a time when you felt a sense of clarity and certainty—about your direction in life, your identity, your relationships, or something equally important. How did you come to be so certain? What values did this certainty reflect?

_____

_____

_____

_____

_____

_____

_____

_____

_____

_____

_____

_____

_____

_____

_____

_____

"Queer millennials are setting the tone and holding society accountable in a way generations before never had the opportunity to. We are emitting a burning necessity and urgency about our journeys."

—*Raquel Willis*

When you're struggling with strong, uncomfortable emotions brought on by life events, it might seem like they're never going to end. However, in the long term, even intense distress eventually fades or lessens in intensity. Keeping this in mind might help you make better decisions.

Write about a strong emotion you experienced last year. How long did it last? What did you do in response? How do you feel about your reaction after you've gained some distance?

Free Yourself From Expectations

Do you ever feel like you're always the one to initiate contact or make plans with other people? This week, set yourself free from these expectations. Allow other people to reach out to you, or ask someone else to plan an outing.

Think about a time when you've blamed or criticized yourself for having a particular problem. If a friend came to you with this problem, how would you advise and comfort them? How would it be different from what you would tell yourself?

_____

_____

_____

_____

_____

_____

_____

_____

_____

_____

_____

_____

_____

_____

_____

_____

Regret is something a lot of trans people experience. Maybe you wish you had come out sooner. Or maybe you envy people who got to make physical changes to their bodies earlier than you did. It's possible to acknowledge regret without having to "fix" it or letting it deter you from future opportunities. Write (without judgment) about a regret you have.

Making Your Voice Heard

Sometimes, trans people hide who they are for important reasons, like safety. At other times, they might do it to preserve their relationships with others, even if it means that they feel unseen and unheard in some ways. This can interfere with how close they are able to feel with friends and family. This week, find a way to show more of who you are to someone you care about.

Moving Beyond Labels

Some people grow up with labels, like "caregiver," "loser," or "prodigy." Often, these labels are tied to gender roles and stereotypes. What are some labels people have assigned you? On the left, write any labels you've been assigned. On the right, write a few words about how well each one fits you.

Example:

Hard Worker   **I wish I were allowed to be lazy!**

_____   _____

_____   _____

_____   _____

_____   _____

_____   _____

_____   _____

_____   _____

_____   _____

Where do you feel like your worth as a person comes from? Is it contained in your social class, career, or net worth? Your accomplishments or contributions to society? If you believe your inherent worth is contingent on external factors—like others' approval, your academic achievements, your finances, or your job—you might feel worthless if you think you don't measure up in any of these domains. This might cause you to feel self-conscious, or to avoid threats to your self-esteem by staying away from challenging tasks that could be rewarding. Write about what makes you a worthwhile person that has nothing to do with external validation or concrete accomplishments.

"Habituation" describes what happens when you're exposed to a scenario so many times that you get used to it. For example, if you have to be assertive with customers at work every day, you might get to a point where you stop feeling anxious about it. Write about a time you developed skills or strength in stressful times.

_____

_____

_____

_____

_____

_____

_____

_____

_____

_____

_____

_____

Stereotypes can affect your willingness to take risks and try new things. For example, you might not want to get an engineering degree because you're worried you'll fail and prove to everyone that people like you aren't cut out for STEM careers. Write about a stereotype that's held you back.

_____

_____

_____

_____

_____

_____

_____

_____

_____

_____

_____

_____

_____

When someone expresses a negative emotion to you, especially if that emotion is about you, it might be tempting to apologize or try to "fix" that emotion, even if you don't feel like you've done anything wrong. This can cause you to sacrifice your happiness for others' comfort—for example, not expressing your identified gender when you go home for Christmas because your parents don't accept it. Write about a time you felt pressured into taking care of someone else's emotions.

Give Yourself a Break

If you have a strong sense of justice, you may feel the urge to respond to every injustice you encounter. Maybe you find yourself jumping into debates in online comment sections or constantly correcting misconceptions about trans people. This week, if you find that fighting injustice has become exhausting, give yourself a break from trying to fix any but the most important, life-or-death injustices.

I can change my mind if I want to. Changing my mind doesn't mean that the feelings I had before weren't valid. Changing my mind means that I'm capable of learning from my experiences and listening to my needs.

Sorry, It's Private

Being trans can feel embarrassingly public. You might feel like you have to answer everyone's questions about your body, identity, or sexuality. But a trans identity isn't a license for people to make you uncomfortable. Practice saying these phrases out loud in the mirror:

- ○ "Sorry, it's private!"
- ○ "I don't talk about that stuff at work."
- ○ "That's a really rude question."
- ○ "I don't feel comfortable answering that."
- ○ "Please don't comment on my body."
- ○ "It's not up for debate."

Responsibility is a scary thing. It can be tempting to blame others for our failures or to believe that others are at fault for holding us back. These feelings can be based in reality, but focusing on the parts of your life you can't control can make it hard to make changes in situations you *can* control. Write about something in your life you feel is within your control.

Asking for help can be a vulnerable experience. It might feel like you're taking resources away from people who need them or opening yourself up to criticism for not being independent enough. It's important to realize that no one is truly independent. Some forms of dependence on others are socially sanctioned (like hiring someone to do your taxes), while others—wrongly—are considered less acceptable (like applying for food stamps if you can't afford groceries). Like it or not, we all rely on other people in some way to help us, heal us, or defend us. Write about the help you need right now and how you can go about asking for it.

_____

_____

_____

_____

_____

_____

_____

_____

_____

_____

_____

_____

_____

_____

Stating Your Needs

Having conversations about your gender with other people can be daunting. It might help you organize your thoughts if you think about these conversations in terms of your needs. Do you need the other person to understand something, do something, or change their behavior in some way? Write about conversations you hope to have in the future.

Example:

I need <u>my friend Cathy</u> **to** <u>include me in girls' nights</u> **so I can feel more** <u>affirmed</u>.

I need _____ to _____

so I can feel more _____.

I need _____ to _____

so I can feel more _____.

I need _____ to _____

so I can feel more _____.

Write about a time you felt fully relaxed and stress-free. What was different about that time?

_____

_____

_____

_____

_____

_____

_____

_____

_____

_____

_____

_____

_____

_____

When you hear the word "selfish," what comes to mind? Many people worry about being selfish anytime they do something small for themselves—even if it's just going to dinner by themselves instead of cooking dinner for their roommates or calling out of a volunteer job when they're feeling run-down. If you're an activist and spend a lot of your time fighting for good causes, it can feel like any time you spend having fun takes away from important work. But having boundaries about how much you're willing to do for others is important, especially if being unselfish is causing you to feel burned out. Write about how you might draw boundaries around the time, money, and energy you spend on yourself.

If all of your problems went away tomorrow, how would you know? When you picture this scenario, you might think about material circumstances, such as your job. But you might also be thinking about your behavior, beliefs, or attitude toward life. Write about the mental and emotional changes that would happen in a perfect world.

_____

_____

_____

_____

_____

_____

_____

_____

_____

_____

_____

_____

_____

Connect with Your Body

Welcome to the hands-on, physical, sweaty section of the book. We're going to build your self-acceptance muscles, pump up your ability to listen to your body's signals, and Jazzercise your physical self-care techniques. (Whew. I might need to do some Strained Metaphor Yoga now.)

In this section, the prompts, quotes, affirmations, and exercises will focus on getting in tune with what your body is telling you. We'll explore not just concrete topics like fitness and stress, but more abstract stuff like body image and self-consciousness. We'll also talk about how these topics relate to gender identity, transition, stereotypes, and being a trans person in the world.

"When people are seen as real, and no longer theoretical, it becomes harder to exclude them."

—Laura Erickson-Schroth
and Laura A. Jacobs

Some trans people carry a lot of tension in their bodies. You might be used to slumping over to hide your chest or crouching down to look less tall. Maybe you're so disconnected from your body that you don't notice pain and discomfort. Write about the physical sensations in your body today, positive and negative. What might you need to make time for—like getting out of your chair, taking an exercise class, or seeing a doctor—that could relieve some of the more negative sensations? And what could you do to bring more of the positive sensations into your life?

If you're not feeling body positive right now, try what's called "body neutrality." Body neutrality means spending less time worrying about how you feel about your appearance, positive or negative. It means putting less emphasis on being "beautiful" or loving your physical features and more on what your body can do: playing an instrument, swimming laps, or just carrying you through your day. Write about the things your body can do that have nothing to do with how you look.

Effortless Fun

Have you ever felt tired and stressed at the end of your day off? Many people find it hard to relax, even with no work, school, or childcare. Maybe you feel like you have to put in more effort than everyone else just to keep up. Or maybe you take on volunteer projects that don't count as "work" to you. Whatever the cause, it's not healthy to go without real breaks. Next time you're free, set aside an hour for an activity that doesn't involve self-improvement, personal projects, or helping people—just effortless fun.

When was the last time you discovered your body could do something you didn't know it was capable of, like running a 5K or overcoming a health problem? Why didn't you think you could do it, and what did you learn about yourself when you found you could?

Taking Up Space

How much space do you take up? Many trans people are afraid of taking up too much. It might be because you'd rather not be noticed by other people, or because you feel like you don't have the right to take up space. Maybe you're worried about inconveniencing other people with the size of your body or the way you get around. Write about how it feels to take up physical space. This week, try these activities to expand your sense of the space you're allowed to take up:

- ○ Do you let people talk over or interrupt you? Keep talking instead of stopping. If necessary, raise your voice.

- ○ Do you always get out of other people's way, even when there's enough space for both of you? Find yourself squeezing past others? Ask if they can make space for you instead.

- ○ Do you take the worst seat or cram yourself into a corner when you're with friends? Take the seat you want.

- ○ Do you try to make yourself smaller in a group? Pick your head up and let your arms and legs relax to a point where they're comfortable.

"[I]n long distance adventure skating, the memories go beyond the board. It's the people who beep and wave at you as you climb a huge hill, it's the cyclists who smile when they see a 30-pound backpack on your person, it's the shop owners who go out of their way to make sure you are fed and comfortable, it's the feeling of taking your backpack off and being soaked in sweat that you earned."

—*Calleigh Little,*
first transgender woman to skateboard
across the United States

Do you need to HALT? HALT reminds you to take a moment to check in and see if you are hungry, angry, lonely, or tired. When you're any of those things, you might feel bad enough to make impulsive decisions or snap at someone. Paying attention to the physical sensations in your body can make you aware of when you need to meet your needs in the moment—be it grabbing a snack if you are hungry, taking five minutes to cool down if you are angry, reaching out to a friend when you feel lonely, or taking a power nap when you are tired. Write down your HALT warning signs:

Hungry (examples: stomach pain, light-headedness, decreased energy, brain fog, shakiness, headache):

_____

_____

Angry (examples: pressure in head or sinus, chest tightness, muscle tension, feeling hot, sweating, difficulty breathing, increased heartbeat):

_____

_____

Lonely (examples: feeling of emptiness, scrolling endlessly on social media):

_____

_____

Tired (examples: drowsiness, irritability, difficulty concentrating):

_____

_____

Have you ever told yourself that you "should" exercise? Say, why *do* people exercise? Is it competition, challenge, or teamwork? Changing your appearance, like lifting weights to get buff? Making everyday tasks like climbing stairs easier? Feeling physically or mentally better? Or just the joy of moving your body?

It can be tough to separate the cultural messages you get about exercise—like "stop being lazy" or "lose weight"—from your internal motivation. It can also be difficult to separate these messages from the expectations of your identified or designated gender, like being curvy or muscular. If you exercise now, write about what motivates you. If you don't, write about what you might like to get out of exercise—for you, not for anyone else.

Are there parts of your body you like that are *not* typical for someone of your identified gender? Write about a piece of you that is gloriously atypical.

_____

_____

_____

_____

_____

_____

_____

_____

_____

_____

_____

_____

_____

_____

_____

_____

Honor Your Body

How do you like to be touched? If you have a partner, you might find it tricky to balance their needs—the way *they* like to be physical with *you*—with your feelings about your body. You might have parts you don't want to show them or ways of touching that don't feel right. Or you might want to be touched in ways that you haven't voiced to them. This week, find a time to talk with your partner about your needs around your physical body. If you don't have a partner, find a time to be assertive about your physical needs in another way—like saying no to a hug or taking a long lunch away from your desk.

I will not get to where I need to be with my body by moving away from discomfort. If I want to run my first marathon, I will have to train consistently. If I want to assert my body's needs around other people, I will have to face social discomfort. If I want to be kinder and more forgiving toward my body, I will have to confront beliefs about myself that may be painful or embarrassing.

You know those movie montages in which someone's trying to get in shape? A few scenes of the character sweating into a tracksuit and lifting a few weights—boom, they're done! Unfortunately for real people, making body changes—whether they are tangible changes, like getting physical therapy, or more abstract changes, like improving your body image—takes time. Write about a change you're working toward that's going slowly. Why is it important to take your time?

We're bombarded with "shoulds" and "musts" about our bodies every day. Turn on your TV and you'll instantly find that you *should* have rock-hard biceps and you *must* watch your sugar intake. But we all have different goals and priorities, which means that nothing is 100 percent imperative for everyone. Try to add some *ifs* to those shoulds.

Examples:

"I should change my eating habits . . . if my doctor identifies that as a health problem for me."

"I should go for a run . . . if my priority right now is to get better at running."

"I should eat fewer calories . . . if I want to lose weight, which is not something I'm obligated to do."

What kinds of changes would I need to feel comfortable in my body? What kind of exploration would help me understand my relationship with my body? These questions can be hard to ask if you're unable to express or explore your gender where you are, or with the people you know. You might feel the need to conform to stereotypes about your designated or identified gender just to get by.

Write about what kind of environment you'd need to get to a better place with your body. Even if it's not possible now, how can you work toward getting there?

This outfit isn't for me. What do you mean when you say that? Sometimes, you're just not feeling plaid today. However, you might also be saying something like:

○ I don't want people to see the shape of my body.

○ I'm afraid to show this aspect of my gender.

○ I don't think I'm the type of person who is allowed to wear this because of my gender, age, or body type.

Write about an outfit you're afraid to wear. Why are you afraid to wear it? And what would it take for you to feel comfortable wearing it?

_____

_____

_____

_____

_____

_____

_____

_____

_____

_____

_____

Getting Comfortable

Ever feel self-conscious about your body? Next time you're in a situation in which you feel overly aware of your physical appearance or behavior, try to dig into why. What are you trying to hide or minimize? Ask yourself:

- How likely is it that people are paying close attention to me?

- Is what I'm self-conscious about really as shameful or unusual as I think it is?

- If someone did think critical thoughts about me, how bad would that be?

- If I mess up or look weird, how long would people actually remember it?

- What are the consequences of letting self-consciousness dictate where I go and what I do?

If you are older, do you feel like age has made you better able to weather changes or stand up for yourself? If you are younger, do you think it gives you more options in life? Write about your relationship with your age.

_____

_____

_____

_____

_____

_____

_____

_____

_____

_____

_____

_____

_____

_____

_____

_____

How do you feel about difficult and daunting tasks? If you were told as a kid that you weren't doing well in school unless you got an effortless A, or if you got cut from track because you weren't improving as quickly as your coach wanted, you might now equate difficulty with inadequacy. The idea that talented people do everything well on the first try can keep you from developing your skills. Write about something difficult you've done and how it's changed your perspective.

Being around certain people might make you feel better about your body than others. You might have friends who talk about themselves positively or validate your self-image struggles, or coworkers who turn every conversation toward celebrities' beach bodies. Write about the people in your life and how they make you feel about your body.

Masturbation can be a great way to figure out your needs around physical pleasure. When you're having sex with yourself, you can tune into the fine points of your own experience without having to worry about a partner or feel self-conscious about your body or performance.

Write down three to four things that make solo sex more pleasurable for you—including less tangible things, like "having more time" or "being able to be as loud as I want." Write down an additional three to four things you might like to try in the future. You might be able to incorporate these factors into partnered sex in the future, or just enjoy them on your own. If masturbation or sex isn't your thing, write about other sensual experiences, like getting a hot stone massage.

Not into fitness? Time to get creative with physical movement. You don't have to play a sport if you want to get fitter—whether that means boosting your endurance, strengthening your muscles, or improving your mobility. What can you do at your job to incorporate more standing, walking, or lifting?

Example: **As a nurse, I can take shifts on a unit where I'll be on my feet more.**

What's something you do for fun that could incorporate more movement?

Example: **I love walking in the park, so maybe I could try some uphill hikes.**

_____

_____

_____

_____

What can you change about your routine that could get you moving more?

Example: **Instead of driving, I could cycle to work.**

_____

_____

_____

If you're the studious type who would like to forget you have a body, it's easy to neglect your physical needs. But the further you go down that road, the more your mood, cognition, and stress levels suffer. Write about some physical needs you need to meet if you want your brain to function at its best. Examples might include prioritizing sleep, eating regular meals, fulfilling your need for physical touch and closeness, or getting medical care you've put off.

_____

_____

_____

Spiritual and religious traditions have a lot to say about the human body. Some traditions teach that your body is an unimportant earthly vessel for your soul. Others, like Buddhism, teach that the body is an essential, interdependent element of one's self. Many religions have rules about what you should and shouldn't do with your body. Write about the relationship between your religion or spirituality—or your family's or community's—and your body.

_____

_____

_____

_____

_____

_____

_____

_____

_____

_____

_____

_____

_____

Unlock Your Creativity

This is what people buy journals for, right? This section is about getting to a place where you can make something great, whether you're mastering the art of bunraku puppetry, learning flair bartending, or trying to revive the lost art of underwater break dancing. (If that exists, please let me know.)

The prompts, quotes, affirmations, and exercises in this section will focus on taking a closer look at your talents. You'll be challenged to reassess your beliefs about your skills, try things you're not sure you'll like, and think carefully about the reasons behind why you create. You'll also look at the ways in which your gender experiences fit into your creative life. Let's go!

"For me, writing online was like shooting a flare into the sky. I wanted those kids to know there was some kind of hope. I hadn't necessarily found it for myself at first, but I really believed we were going to find it together."

—Sam Dylan Finch

What's something you're not good at, but love to do anyway? Think Linda Belcher's off-key singing in *Bob's Burgers*, or Elaine Benes's dancing in *Seinfeld*. Maybe it's an "unflattering" outfit you rock to brunch, or a truly terrible novel you've only shown your best friend. Write about your guilty passion. What is it, and why doesn't it matter that you're bad at it?

It's easy to delay creative projects until things are "perfect," like waiting to get a burst of inspiration and an entire Saturday of free time to start your next play. Maybe you're waiting until after you've completed a physical transition goal or reached some milestone, like moving to a new city. Whatever your medium, it might be time to strike a balance between setting lofty goals and allowing yourself to be creative where you are now. Write about a creative work you've been putting off. What are some fun, low-pressure steps you can take to get started?

"When it comes to performance art, I am more interested in the failures than the so-called successes. I have never cared for entertaining anyone. My performances may have elements that some may find entertaining, but that's not my main purpose. If you want pure entertainment value just go and see something like Stomp or Blue Man Group."

—*Vaginal Davis*

Creativity is an end in itself. My work doesn't have to be on display in a gallery or published in a book to be valuable.

Showing someone your work puts you in a vulnerable position. On one hand, you might get crucial feedback or affirmation that you're going in the right direction. On the other, you might hear things that are painful to hear—even if they end up being valuable to you. Write about your relationship with vulnerability as it relates to your creative work.

You know how they say, "Everyone's a critic"? Not everyone's the right critic for you. Some people are so close to you that they can't be objective. Others might know nothing about your medium or be terrible at organizing their thoughts. Write about exactly the kind of feedback you need on your work.

_____

_____

_____

_____

_____

_____

_____

_____

_____

_____

_____

_____

_____

_____

_____

Trans characters in media can open up your sense of possibility, especially when you're still figuring things out. Maybe the first trans person you read about was a character in a novel. Maybe seeing a nonbinary person on TV when you've only known binary trans people in real life makes you feel seen. Write about why representation is important to you, either in your own creative work or in the work you appreciate.

Play can help you break through creative blocks. When you play, you don't have to commit to anything serious. You can play with words without feeling obligated to write a whole novel, or dance without having to choreograph your magnum opus.

What's something fun and noncommittal you can do with your chosen medium?

Example: **A short, just-for-laughs poem if you consider yourself a poet.**

_____

_____

_____

_____

_____

_____

_____

How might you play by using your chosen medium in a different way?

Example: **Writing fiction if you're a nonfiction writer.**

_____

_____

_____

_____

How can you play with gender in your creative endeavors? What are some unserious ways you can explore your identity?

Novelist Jenny Offill coined the term "art monster": someone who joyfully neglects their responsibilities to create art. Gender often has to do with whether you're allowed to be an art monster. As Offill writes in the novel *Dept. of Speculation,* "Women almost never become art monsters because art monsters only concern themselves with art, never mundane things. Nabokov didn't even fold his umbrella. Véra licked his stamps for him." If you're a woman, feminine person, or were designated female at birth, gender roles might get in the way of your carving out space between your mundane responsibilities to create art. Write about how you might enhance your art-monstering capabilities.

Who are your creative heroes? Thinking about our favorite artists and writers can spur us to go deeper in our own work. It can be even more illuminating to think about the ones with whom we share important differences. What are the common factors? Let's find out.

Who's your favorite creative outside your favorite genre? What draws you in about them despite not usually being into that type of work?

_____

_____

_____

_____

Who's your favorite creative with whom you have a love/hate relationship? What makes you like some of their work, but not others?

_____

_____

_____

_____

Who's your favorite creative whose life experiences or identity differs drastically from yours? Why does their work reach you across that divide?

_____

_____

_____

_____

Psychiatrist and Holocaust survivor Viktor Frankl once wrote that: "If there is a meaning in life at all, then there must be a meaning in suffering." Sometimes, misery is just misery. But you don't have to "make the best" of your troubles or "look on the bright side" to see meaning in the sad or scary things that have happened to you, or to find creative purpose in dark times. Write about the ways in which suffering has led to creativity for you.

Creative Constraints

Constraints can help you get out of creative ruts. If you find yourself returning to the same themes or type of work in your creative endeavors, it might be time to give yourself some artificial limits so that you can wear a new groove with your work. This week, put a constraint on one of your projects, like making your new short story a long letter or writing a song without using the word "the."

Perfectionism can be useful when you're finishing a project, but being afraid of failure might prevent you from even starting one. Write about your relationship with perfection. How has perfection helped you or held you back? What's your ideal balance between quality and quantity?

_____

_____

_____

_____

_____

_____

_____

_____

_____

_____

_____

_____

_____

_____

_____

Passion Projects

Do you schedule time for creative projects, or do you work on art in the margins of your life? If you only create when you have nothing else to do, your productivity is probably suffering. This week, create specific time blocks on your calendar to work on passion projects.

What if you don't consider yourself a creative person? You might have looked at some of these prompts and said, "I'm not a prolific writer or a passionate filmmaker. What's my place in all this?" But creativity can show up in unexpected places—like coming up with a novel solution to a tough problem or buying the perfect gift. Write about your everyday creativity.

_____

_____

_____

_____

_____

_____

_____

_____

_____

_____

_____

_____

_____

A Few Ideas...

Starting a creative hobby can be overwhelming. Who knew a spinning wheel was so expensive or that oil painting classes were so time-consuming? But after a long day of work meetings and a long evening of scrubbing your shower, you're desperate for some stress relief. Here are some low-cost, low-stakes ways of getting creative.

Painting and drawing: Mixed media can save a lot of money on materials. Many artists use unusual (and cheap!) materials like ballpoint pens, magazine cutouts, bubble wrap, and yarn. What can you make with what you have on hand?

Writing and poetry: If you're intimidated by a blank page, use someone else's words. Cut some words and phrases out of newspapers or use an online random word generator to get your story started. Borrow a phrase from your favorite book as an opening line. Or try blackout poetry: buy a book from a thrift store and color over all of the words except the ones you want to use for your poem.

Culinary arts: Give yourself a grocery store challenge. What can you create for $5, $10, or $20? Can you whip cream, cocoa powder, and sugar into chocolate mousse? Can those bruised apples and discount berries be turned into fruit wine? Can you make a decadent hot pot feast or taco dinner for friends on a limited budget?

Photography: Have you really *seen* your town or city? I bet there are local landmarks you've never looked twice at—a covered bridge, a famous mountain, or even just a weird house you've never seen up close. Get up close and personal with your phone or camera. Try different times of day or different filters or effects.

What's your niche? Trying to make your creative work accessible or relatable for a mainstream audience might dilute the quality, cause you to censor yourself, or drive you nuts with anxiety about bad reviews. This might also be true of the things you do at your job, in your hobbies, or in your life in general. Maybe you didn't want to propose a new project at work because you were afraid your coworkers might criticize it, or you were worried about what your in-laws would say about that daring living room makeover you wanted. Write about the kind of things you'd do—in your creative work, or just in life—if you didn't worry about success or popularity.

_____

_____

_____

_____

_____

_____

_____

_____

_____

_____

_____

_____

_____

Being trans sometimes means having to get creative in unexpected situations. Have you ever made a binder out of an old pair of tights or spent days thinking up the perfect chosen name? Write about ways your gender identity or expression has caused you to get creative.

_____

_____

_____

_____

_____

_____

_____

_____

_____

_____

_____

_____

_____

Think about the first time you can remember showing an adult something you'd made as a kid. What did they say? If it was helpful or affirming, write about that. If it wasn't, write about what it taught you about the kind of feedback you need.

_____

_____

_____

_____

_____

_____

_____

_____

_____

_____

_____

_____

_____

_____

_____

Draw a self-portrait in the space that follows. It could be the way you see yourself, the way other people see you, or something else altogether. It doesn't have to look like you—or look like anything.

Hidden Talents

Think about yourself a year ago. What have you learned about your creative passions or skills that you'd love to tell your slightly-more-clueless self? Have you discovered a talent for cooking after your favorite takeout place closed or found yourself drawn to portraits after years of photographing landscapes? Sharpened a skill just by devoting more time to it? And with that in mind, what do you think you'll need to do in the coming year to further hone your skills or explore your passions?

Artistic Allies

Who are your creative allies? The people who listen to your wildest fan fiction ideas, or pose for yet another photo series? This week, do some thinking about the kind of network you need to create what you're meant to create. If you feel you don't have enough creative allies, how do you think you might build that support? Or if you have enough, how can you support others in their creativity?

For some people, their creative work reflects their real, honest selves better than anything else. How does your work reflect you? What's inside you that you'd like to reveal to other people when they see your work?

_____

_____

_____

_____

_____

_____

_____

_____

_____

_____

_____

_____

_____

_____

_____

Write a 10-word biography of yourself.

_____

_____

_____

_____

_____

_____

_____

Now circle the most important descriptor of yourself. Why is it important?

_____

_____

_____

_____

_____

_____

Surround Yourself with a Supportive Community

There's a reason they call it "the trans community" instead of "the trans just-you-sitting-in-front-of-your-TV-with-your-cat." You need people in your corner who affirm you: trans people who know exactly where you're coming from and cis allies who get what it means to support you. Caring for yourself means being discerning about who you let into your life and what boundaries you set with them.

This section is about the way we give and get support. Even the most independent person in the world can't make it without other people—whether it's your dad who takes you to your therapy appointments, your church friends who turned up to the protest with markers and cardboard, or your well-intentioned coworkers who misspelled your chosen name on the company birthday card. The prompts, exercises, quotes, and affirmations in this section will focus on how to build a community you can rely on when you need it.

"If I wait for someone else to validate my existence, it will mean that I'm shortchanging myself."

—Zanele Muholi

What are friends for? No, really—what *do* you need in a friend? If you've ever found yourself getting so focused on getting someone to like you that you forgot whether your own needs were getting met, you may not have ever considered what *you'd* like to have in a friend. Do you need someone who's honest to the point of bluntness? Sensitive to your boundaries? Trustworthy with your secrets? Write about your ideal friend.

If you're on the independent end of the spectrum, you might feel uncomfortable relying on other people or letting them rely on you, even when it means going without something you need. Like it or not, we're all interdependent—unless you're living in a cave and growing your own vegetables by candlelight. Write about a time when your fate was unexpectedly intertwined with someone else's. How did it change the situation so that you were able to depend on someone or let someone depend on you? Were there any unexpected benefits?

_____

_____

_____

_____

_____

_____

_____

_____

_____

_____

_____

_____

_____

Write about a conversation you've had that has affirmed your identity. What made it so supportive? Based on your feelings about this conversation, what kind of support do you feel you need?

_____

_____

_____

_____

_____

_____

_____

_____

_____

_____

_____

_____

_____

_____

We tend to associate queer and trans communities with gathering spaces, like LGBTQ community centers and support groups. But you might have built a community in an entirely different way—maybe in your place of worship, your workplace, or online. Write about the interesting places where you've found community.

_____

_____

_____

_____

_____

_____

_____

_____

_____

_____

_____

_____

_____

"Like racism and all forms of prejudice, bigotry against transgender people is a deadly carcinogen. We are pitted against each other in order to keep us from seeing each other as allies. Genuine bonds of solidarity can be forged between people who respect each other's differences and are willing to fight their enemy together. We are the class that does the work of the world, and can revolutionize it."

—Leslie Feinberg

When you were a kid, you could be friends with anyone who shared half an ice pop with you. What changed? What do you need now that you didn't need as a kid? Different kinds of support? People who share your experiences? Important similarities or differences? Write about how your childhood or teenage friends are different from the friends you have now.

Healthy Boundaries

Have you ever heard someone say, "I'd do anything for my friends"? In reality, everyone has limits that even their close friends can't cross. If you find yourself making exceptions to your personal rules because you're worried people will get mad at you or feel hurt, you might have a problem with boundaries.

In the blank spaces, write about the rules you set for others.

Even my close friends can't ask me for _____

_____.

I don't let people say _____

_____ to me.

If a friend did _____

_____, we'd have

to have a serious conversation.

I used to think it was okay for people to _____

_____,

but now I speak up when it happens.

How do you feel like you fit into your local trans or queer community? Fitting in isn't just being around people who share your experiences. Maybe the people in your local community are so similar that it's an echo chamber in there. Or maybe your community is so inclusive that it ends up including people who make everyone *else* feel excluded. Or maybe it's great and you feel like you've found your people. Write about your local trans/queer community and how you fit in. Or, if you don't feel like you fit in, write about what would help you feel more comfortable.

Relationship therapists Drs. Julie and John Gottman often talk about "rituals of connection": habits and rituals that you share with your partner to build trust and intimacy. We can build these rituals in nonromantic relationships, too. What are some rituals of connection you share with friends and family—like a board game night you never miss or a bad gift that keeps getting regifted to different family members every Christmas?

In *The Simpsons* episode "The Old Man and the 'C' Student," Bart Simpson is forced to do community service at the Springfield Retirement Castle. By the time his community service hours are up, he's become so attached to the residents that he decides to keep volunteering. Write about a place you didn't think you'd find community, but did.

Assuming you haven't been in a coma since the early 2000s, being friends with someone means figuring out how they fit into your social media sphere. Just because you like someone doesn't mean you need to know every time they buy a new cereal, and you may not be ready to share details about a death in your family with Friendly Coworker Bob.

In the following space, in the left-hand column, write some the names of people whom you'd feel comfortable reading your innermost thoughts. In the middle column, write some names of people you'd show cute dog pics, but not the heavy stuff. In the right-hand column, write the names of people you don't want in your social media at all. Take some time this week to go through your profiles and make adjustments to your privacy settings if you've accidentally let a "cute dog photos only" person into your "innermost thoughts" circle.

Closest Contacts	"Cute Dog Pics" List	Unfollow List

As a therapist, I've lost count of the number of times someone has told me that they don't feel "trans enough." Sometimes, it's because they don't fit into binary gender stereotypes, or look like what they think a "real" trans person looks like. Or it might be because they haven't gone past some arbitrary milestone, like getting gender-affirming medical treatment or "figuring out" their gender once and for all. I often find that these clients feel much more sure of themselves when they see trans people who look like them or who have struggled with those same thoughts. Write about a time you felt that you saw yourself in another trans person.

What have you let go of this year? A romantic relationship that wasn't working out, a community that didn't feel right, or a friendship that didn't support you in quite the right way? Or maybe it was something more abstract, like needing someone's approval or wanting to reconnect with someone who wasn't good for you. Write a breakup letter to someone or something you let go of this year.

_____

_____

_____

_____

_____

_____

_____

_____

_____

_____

_____

_____

_____

_____

"Attribution" is a psychology term used to describe people's beliefs about why things happen and why people do the things they do. Our assumptions about other people's behavior shape the way we feel about them. For example, if you don't like someone, you might assume that they posted a photo of their expensive vacation on Instagram just to make you feel jealous. Assuming the worst about people's intentions can prevent you from forming trusting relationships with others.

In the following space, write about a negative assumption you made about someone's intentions or motives, and come up with some possible alternative explanations for their behavior.

Assumption:

_____

_____

Possible explanations:

_____

_____

Assumption:

_____

_____

Possible explanations:

_____

_____

There is a community out there filled with people who will support and accept me. It may take time to find, but it'll be worth it. I'm worthy of friendship and respect even if I haven't yet found my people.

Write about a time you collaborated with other people on a project. What did you create? How was it different from something you created solo?

_____

_____

_____

_____

_____

_____

This month, when you're looking for an opportunity to socialize or volunteer, look outside your normal circles, such as a new group where you're not sure you'd fit in or a nonprofit in a far-off neighborhood. Jot down any ideas you might already have.

_____

_____

_____

_____

_____

_____

_____

Write about what kinds of relationships you hope to have cultivated a year from now. What will you need to change in order for that to happen?

"I feel like I was like a
little turtle inside the little shell,
and now I'm just like a full blown,
like . . . what's not a turtle?"

—Aja

Ever draw a picture of your family in school as a kid? Here's your chance to bring that picture up to date. Your chosen family is the circle of people you've deliberately brought into your life to love, support, and affirm you—whether they're related to you or came into your life in a different way. Draw or collage your chosen family in the space that follows.

Hallmark movies would have you believe that relationships that don't last forever aren't worth having. But even short-term friendship—a college roommate who changed your perspective or a community theater group you still think about even though it's been years—can be meaningful. Write about someone (or a group of people) you knew for a short time who changed you.

How much of yourself do you feel you can show the people around you? Hiding aspects of yourself—especially something core to you, like your gender identity or sexuality—can make you feel like the "you" people like isn't actually you. It's hard to cultivate intimacy without vulnerability, which may mean showing people aspects of yourself that you're scared to show. Write about an aspect of yourself you're afraid to let others see. What would need to change for you to be able to show that side to others?

True Friends?

It can be difficult to recognize abuse and manipulation outside of romantic relationships. That friend who's always "playfully" putting you down or getting in your physical space doesn't necessarily fit into the stereotypes we hold about abuse. Worse, emotional manipulation may make you feel like *you're* the one in the wrong. If you're second-guessing yourself about a friendship, take this quiz. Check any box that reflects how you feel.

○ I feel bad when I'm around them, but I can't figure out why.

○ I don't feel like I can ever say no to them.

○ They blame me for their behavior.

○ They've never apologized to me, but I'm always apologizing to them.

○ They downplay their behavior or outright say it didn't happen.

○ They say they're "joking" after they do something mean.

○ They've threatened to do something drastic when I've reduced contact with them.

○ They get other friends to gang up on me.

○ I always feel guilty around them, but I can't think of anything specific I did wrong.

○ I feel like I'll never be good enough for them to respect me, no matter how hard I try.

If you checked even one of these boxes, it might be worth taking some time away from this friendship to see how you feel after a little distance. (And if you don't feel like you're "allowed" to get some distance from this friendship, that should tell you something important, too.)

What do you have to offer others? Write about what you have to give as a friend or community member. Try to think about qualities you have (e.g., honesty) or emotional support you can offer (e.g., encouragement) rather than concrete things you can do for others (e.g., helping them move).

In high school, getting rejected by a potential friend might have been devastating. As an adult, you've likely started to realize that you can be the world's greatest person and still not be compatible with someone. In fact, you've probably learned to be a bit more discerning yourself.

In the inner circle that follows, write a few of your "must-haves": characteristics and behaviors that potential friends absolutely need to have. In the outer circle, write a few of your "nice-to-haves": the stuff you can be flexible about.

Embrace Your Authentic Self

Who *are* you? If you've ever hesitated to answer that question—maybe because you're embarrassed or ashamed of the answer, or afraid of others' reactions—this section is for you. The prompts, exercises, quotes, and affirmations in this section are all about accepting and celebrating every facet of yourself, pushing back against norms, claiming the space you need, and fighting shame and stigma.

"Queer people don't grow up as ourselves, we grow up playing a version of ourselves that sacrifices authenticity to minimize humiliation and prejudice. The massive task of our adult lives is to unpick which parts of ourselves are truly us and which parts we've created to protect us. It's massive and existential and difficult. But I'm convinced that being confronted with the need for profound self-discovery so explicitly (and often early in life!) is a gift in disguise."

—Alexander Leon

What did you hide from your family growing up? Having secrets—like a hidden fort in the woods or a kiss you never told anyone about—is a normal part of being a kid. But some of the things we hide reveal deeper truths about us. If you were made to feel uncomfortable about your identity, you may still carry the shame of hiding who you are into adulthood. Write about something you hid from your family that still carries meaning today. What do you wish you could have told your younger self?

Internalized Transphobia

"Internalized transphobia" is a phrase used to describe when people feel shame about their trans identities. Sometimes this manifests itself in self-hatred or blaming oneself for others' prejudices. Other times, it can take the form of looking down on people with different, less socially acceptable trans identities. This week, notice when any feelings of shame related to your identity come up. Try to think about where they come from. Where did you first hear those messages? What have you learned since you first started believing these things about others or yourself?

Have you ever been told to "smile more"? Did it actually make you want to smile? Probably not. Write about a time when someone told you to change the way you express emotion. How did it make you feel, and what do you wish you'd said then?

_____

_____

_____

_____

_____

_____

_____

_____

_____

_____

_____

_____

_____

_____

Do you feel like you aren't where you "should" be in life? Maybe you're seeing glamorous queer people on social media wearing shoes that cost your entire rent check or friends getting gender-affirming healthcare while you lack health insurance. You might blame yourself for these supposed failings or assume you haven't hustled enough to deserve them.

Think about what that means for your mental health. Do you think other people deserve more out of life because they were born into different circumstances? Does it sound fair that some people are less deserving of basic needs, like food and housing? In this quiz, circle the numbers that best represent your feelings.

1. If I haven't worked hard enough, I don't feel like I deserve to feel secure.

2. It's unrealistic to expect me to work 50 hours a week just to stay afloat.

3. I tie a lot of my value to my social status.

4. I don't think it's fair that I or others can't get the healthcare we need.

5. I feel inadequate when I don't meet the usual standards of success.

6. There's nothing wrong with me. It's structural inequality that's wrong.

7. Being in debt is shameful to me.

8. I don't have to be financially successful to have value.

If you picked more odd-numbered answers, you might want to take a hard look at the relationship between your self-worth and your economic status. There's a decent chance that the way you think about success is causing you feelings of shame, stigma, and insecurity.

"Gaslighting" refers to an attempt to persuade someone that their perceptions aren't real. It is a term that was coined by the 1938 play *Gas Light,* in which a husband manipulates and undermines his wife, to the point of convincing her that the gas lamps in their home aren't really dimming—it's just her imagination. (Needless to say, he's the one dimming the lamps.) How did you hold on to your sense of reality?

How can you be flexible with yourself today? Write about the ways you can be gentle on yourself if things don't go according to plan.

_____

_____

_____

_____

_____

_____

_____

_____

_____

_____

_____

_____

_____

_____

_____

Write about a time someone saw something in you that you didn't see in yourself. Perhaps someone in your life recognized a strength you didn't know you had or a piece of yourself you'd tried to hide. What did they see? How did it contribute to your understanding of who you are?

"I have to fight with all my strength to contribute the few positive things my health allows me to the revolution."

—*Frida Kahlo*

Standing up for myself or someone else in the moment is hard. If I don't find exactly the right words, or if those words catch in my throat, I won't beat myself up. Soon, my voice will be heard.

Trans Trailblazers

What do you know about trans history? Seeing yourself represented in history could plant a seed of self-discovery for you. Spend some time researching a notable figure in trans history. Extra points for lesser-known trans pioneers. Mainstream historians tend to ignore trans people with marginalized identities, so you might not find them on Wikipedia. Andrea Jenkins's Tretter Transgender Oral History Project is a great place to start: Lib.umn.edu/tretter/transgender-oral-history-project.

Envy can make you feel small or inadequate, but it can also tell you a lot about yourself. Write about a time you felt envious of someone else's life or accomplishments. What does that tell you about where you need to go in the future?

_____

_____

_____

_____

_____

_____

_____

_____

_____

_____

_____

_____

_____

_____

_____

Being truthful with yourself sometimes means admitting that certain things about you will never change. Are you forgetful? Stubborn? Chronically unfashionable? Write about a flaw—or something you once saw as a flaw—that you've come to accept in yourself.

_____

_____

_____

_____

_____

_____

_____

_____

_____

_____

_____

_____

_____

_____

_____

Where's your comfort zone? We've talked about going outside comfortable places to build assertiveness and distress-tolerance skills. However, sometimes your comfort zone is a place where you relax and renew your energy. Write about what's so comfortable about your comfort zone. How does it help you recharge so that you have more energy for *un*comfortable activities?

_____

_____

_____

_____

_____

_____

_____

_____

_____

_____

_____

_____

_____

_____

Speaking Out

If you've ever read a story about a trans person in a newspaper, you'll notice that journalists often get things wrong. You may have noticed that these stories refer to someone's trans status unnecessarily, make derogatory references to trans people's bodies, or contain phrases like "back when she was a man." Journalism researcher Thomas J. Billard calls this "delegitimizing language": using language that suggests that trans identities are not valid or that trans people are lesser. Self-care for you may mean giving a name to this type of language rather than accepting or ignoring it.

The next time you come across a news story that features a trans person, note where you see delegitimizing language. If you'd like, make a comment or write a letter to the editor. You can find a guide to delegitimizing language here: ThomasJBillard.com/legitimacy-indicators.

Anxiety can feel productive. After all, if you're worrying about something happening in your life or in the world, it's almost like *doing* something! After a long day of anxiety, though, you might be exhausted without getting anything accomplished. Write about things you can do instead of worrying, like making a plan to take action or resting your body so that you can tackle the problem later.

_____

_____

_____

_____

_____

_____

_____

_____

_____

_____

_____

_____

Respect Your Journey

Seeing so many out trans people in the media talking about their lives and identities might make you feel pressured to spill everything about your own gender journey, or to represent the trans community publicly, even if you'd rather keep to yourself. Respecting your own privacy—and accepting that this doesn't necessarily reflect a sense of shame about your identity—is an important part of self-care. What are some parts of your life or identity as a trans person that are private? How can you live authentically *and* maintain boundaries around your personal life?

As a therapist, my clients often tell me that they feel pressured to be grateful. How can they be unsatisfied or unhappy when they have [insert good stuff here]? While gratitude won't necessarily make you instantly happy, feelings of dissatisfaction can often point to unfulfilled wishes and goals. Maybe you have enough material comforts but don't feel a sense of connection with others. Or perhaps you're surrounded by friends and family but lack direction in life. What is your ungratefulness telling you? Why aren't you satisfied with what you have?

What are your strengths as a helper? As you come to better know who you are and where you fit in to your community, your next step might be helping others out. However, you might struggle to do this in a way that honors your abilities. Identifying your strengths and weaknesses can allow you to channel your helping energies in productive ways rather than spinning your wheels when helping in ways that exhaust or discourage you. Maybe you're a great organizer, a talented musician, a fundraiser, or a healer. Write about your helping strengths.

How would your life get better if you were 10 percent more vocal when something bothered you? What about 20 percent? Or 80 percent? Write about what this might change in your life.

_____

_____

_____

_____

_____

_____

_____

_____

_____

_____

_____

_____

_____

_____

_____

Getting healthcare while trans can be an affirming experience or a horrible one. Next time you have to get physical or mental healthcare, go prepared. Under the first prompt below, write at least one question you have for your provider. Under the second, write something your provider can do to make you more comfortable. Under the third, write one thing you can do to make yourself heard during your appointment.

Question for my provider:

_____

_____

_____

I will feel more comfortable if my provider can:

_____

_____

_____

I can make myself heard by:

_____

_____

_____

Telling the truth is inherently empowering. Write about a truth you haven't voiced to anyone yet. In what ways would it be important or freeing to get that truth out?

_____

_____

_____

_____

_____

_____

_____

_____

_____

_____

_____

_____

_____

_____

_____

_____

Think about goals you've put aside for other concerns—like your partner's goals or family problems you had to help with. What can you do today to revisit those goals and make a plan to achieve them?

Your voice is your most powerful tool. Write about a time you've raised your voice—in real life, on paper, or online.

_____

_____

_____

_____

_____

_____

_____

_____

_____

_____

_____

_____

_____

_____

_____

_____

Insight into your goals, barriers, and strengths is one thing—but how do you translate that into action? What are some self-care changes you'd like to make in your life as a result of the things you've learned about yourself?

What do you feel capable of accomplishing today?

_____

_____

_____

_____

What can you do this month for yourself?

_____

_____

_____

_____

What's the most important thing your self-care skills can help you accomplish this year?

_____

_____

_____

_____

RESOURCES

Reading this book may have brought up some powerful emotions. If you're looking to seek the help of a therapist or other professional, these resources may be of help:

TransCareSite.org and **TransHealthcare.org** maintain updated listings of trans-competent healthcare providers, including mental health professionals.

The World Professional Association for Transgender Health (WPATH) has a provider directory (at wpath.org /provider/search) that lists over 100 therapists, as well as primary care doctors, surgeons, and other providers who are members of that organization—myself included!

Psychology Today (PsychologyToday.com), **GoodTherapy** (GoodTherapy.org), and TherapyDen (TherapyDen.com) list therapists who are currently accepting clients and allow you to filter by therapists who specialize in gender identity, are trans-friendly, and/or have lived trans experience.

The organization **GLMA** (glma.org) maintains a provider directory with healthcare providers who have identified themselves as LGBTQ-friendly.

If you are experiencing a crisis or suicidal thoughts, crisis hotlines can help. Call the **Trans Lifeline** (staffed with trans peer counselors only) at 1-877-565-8860 (US) or 1-877-330-6366 (Canada), the **Trevor Project** at 1-866-488-7386 (or text START to 678-678, or visit TheTrevor Project.org for chat support), or the **LGBT National Help Center** at 1-888-843-4564 (or visit glbthotline.org for email and chat support).

ACKNOWLEDGMENTS

I gratefully acknowledge the support of my fellow queer and trans therapists, my partner, Sam, and my editor at Callisto, Adrian Potts. I'm thankful for my clients and the insight they bring to every session. I condemn the actions of my dog, Broccoli, who attempted to eat my glasses during the writing of this book.

ABOUT THE AUTHOR

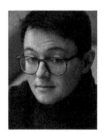 **Andrew Maxwell Triska**, LCSW, is an individual, family, and couples' therapist in New York whose practice focuses on queer and trans clients. Originally from Oregon, Andrew received his education at Williams College (BA), Hunter College (MSW), and New York University (post-master's program in child and family therapy). His experience includes a wide range of work in New York's hospitals, clinics, and nonprofits. Outside of the office, Andrew is a distance runner, a fiction writer, and the author of the *Gender Identity Workbook for Teens*. He is proud to be a trans-identified clinician. His practice can be found online at AndrewTriska.com.

CPSIA information can be obtained
at www.ICGtesting.com
Printed in the USA
JSHW012000170621
16003JS00002B/12

9 781648 763182